15 PATHS

TO

LONG LIFE

Discover the choices to achieving longevity and well-being

Dr. CHARLES A. WOOD

2023 by Dr. Charles A. Wood

Table of contents

INTRODUCTION 4

Chapter 1: Mindful Living 7

Chapter 2: Nutrient-Rich Diets 11

Chapter 3: Regular Exercise 15

Chapter 4: Adequate Sleep 19

Chapter 5: Social Connections 23

Chapter 6: Healthy Aging 29

Chapter 7: Genetics and Epigenetics 33

Chapter 8: Stress Management 39

Chapter 9: Continuous Learning 43

Chapter 10: Purpose and Passion 49

Chapter 11: Traditional Medicine and Alternative Therapies......................55

Chapter 12: Environmental Harmony 63

Chapter 13: Healthy Habits 69

Chapter 14: Financial Wellness 75

Chapter 15: Technology and Longevity............................81

Conclusion...88

INTRODUCTION

In the pursuit of longevity, individuals across cultures and generations have sought various avenues to enhance and extend their lives. The quest for a long and healthy life has inspired diverse practices, habits, and philosophies aimed at promoting well-being and resilience. "50 Paths to Long Life" delves into this rich tapestry of approaches, offering insights into the multifaceted ways people navigate the journey towards a prolonged and fulfilling existence. From traditional wisdom to modern scientific discoveries, this exploration illuminates the diverse pathways individuals have treaded in their aspirations for a life well-lived. Join us on this journey through 50 distinct avenues that encapsulate the collective human endeavor to unlock the secrets of longevity and vitality.

Chapter 1: Mindful Living

Explore the power of mindfulness, stress reduction, and mental well-being as key components for a longer, healthier life.

1.   Definition:

•   Mindful living involves being fully present in the moment, paying attention to thoughts and feelings without judgment.

2.   Awareness:

•   Cultivate awareness of the present moment, focusing on sensations, emotions, and surroundings.

3.   Mind-Body Connection:

•   Recognize the interconnectedness of mind and body, understanding how mental states influence physical well-being.

4.   Breath Awareness:

•   Utilize mindful breathing as a tool to anchor oneself to the present, promoting relaxation and reducing stress.

5.   Non-Judgmental Observation:

•   Observe thoughts and feelings without labeling them as good or bad, fostering a non-judgmental attitude towards oneself.

6.   Acceptance:

• Embrace experiences, both positive and negative, with acceptance, allowing for a more balanced and resilient mindset.

7.   Present-Moment Focus:

• Shift focus from past regrets or future anxieties to the current moment, appreciating the richness of now.

8.   Mindful Eating:

• Practice awareness during meals, savoring each bite, and paying attention to the sensory experience of eating.

9.   Gratitude:

• Cultivate a sense of gratitude for the small moments and aspects of life, promoting a positive outlook.

10.   Stress Reduction:

• Use mindfulness as a stress reduction tool, breaking down overwhelming situations into manageable components.

11.   Emotional Regulation:

• Develop the ability to respond to emotions in a measured way, rather than reacting impulsively.

12.   Mindful Listening:

• Engage in active, mindful listening in conversations, fostering deeper connections with others.

13.   Mindful Movement (Yoga, Tai Chi, etc.):

•   Incorporate mindful movement practices into daily routines, connecting the body and mind through intentional physical activity.

14.   Digital Detox:

•   Take breaks from technology, practicing mindfulness in real-life interactions rather than being constantly connected.

15.   Mindful Work:

•   Apply mindfulness to the workplace, enhancing focus, productivity, and overall job satisfaction.

16.   Self-Compassion:

•   Treat oneself with kindness and understanding, recognizing that everyone faces challenges and imperfections.

17.   Mindful Communication:

•   Communicate with awareness, choosing words intentionally and listening actively to promote understanding.

18.   Nature Connection:

•   Spend time in nature, appreciating the beauty and tranquility it offers, fostering a sense of interconnectedness.

19.   Mindful Sleep:

•	Establish bedtime routines that promote relaxation and mindfulness, improving the quality of sleep.

20.	Continuous Practice:

•	Mindful living is a continuous practice, requiring ongoing effort and a commitment to staying present in all aspects of life.

Chapter 2: Nutrient-Rich Diets

Discover the importance of balanced nutrition, superfoods, and dietary habits that promote longevity.

1.   Balanced Nutrition:

•   Emphasize a well-balanced diet that includes a variety of food groups, providing essential nutrients for overall health.

2.   Colorful Plate:

•   Aim for a colorful plate by incorporating a diverse range of fruits and vegetables, each color indicating different nutrient profiles.

3.   Whole Foods:

•   Prioritize whole, minimally processed foods over highly processed and refined options for maximum nutritional benefit.

4.   Macronutrients:

•   Ensure a balance of macronutrients – carbohydrates, proteins, and fats – to meet energy needs and support bodily functions.

5.   Micronutrients:

• Include a variety of micronutrient-rich foods to obtain essential vitamins and minerals crucial for various physiological processes.

6.   Hydration:

• Stay adequately hydrated with water, as it is vital for digestion, nutrient absorption, and overall bodily functions.

7.   Lean Proteins:

• Incorporate lean protein sources such as poultry, fish, beans, and legumes to support muscle health and repair.

8.   Healthy Fats:

• Choose sources of healthy fats, like avocados, nuts, seeds, and olive oil, for heart health and nutrient absorption.

9.   Fiber-Rich Foods:

• Include high-fiber foods like whole grains, fruits, and vegetables to support digestion, regulate blood sugar, and promote satiety.

10.   Portion Control:

• Practice portion control to maintain a healthy weight and prevent overconsumption of calories.

11.   Limit Added Sugars:

•   Minimize the intake of added sugars, opting for naturally sweet foods and beverages in moderation.

12.   Omega-3 Fatty Acids:

•   Incorporate sources of omega-3 fatty acids, such as fatty fish, flaxseeds, and walnuts, for heart and brain health.

13.   Calcium-Rich Foods:

•   Include dairy or fortified plant-based alternatives, along with leafy greens, for adequate calcium intake to support bone health.

14.   Iron-Rich Foods:

•   Consume iron-rich foods, like lean meats, beans, and leafy greens, to prevent deficiencies and support oxygen transport in the body.

15.   Vitamin D Sources:

•   Ensure sufficient vitamin D intake through sunlight exposure, fortified foods, or supplements to support bone health.

16.   Antioxidant-Rich Choices:

•	Choose foods high in antioxidants, such as berries, dark chocolate, and green tea, to combat oxidative stress and support immune function.

17.	Meal Timing:

•	Distribute meals and snacks throughout the day to maintain steady energy levels and support metabolism.

18.	Individualized Nutrition:

•	Consider individual dietary needs, preferences, and any specific health conditions when planning nutrient-rich meals.

19.	Diverse Protein Sources:

•	Explore diverse protein sources, including plant-based options like tofu, lentils, and quinoa, to enhance nutrient variety.

20.	Consultation with a Nutritionist:

•	Seek guidance from a nutritionist or healthcare professional for personalized advice and to address specific dietary concerns.

Chapter 3: Regular Exercise

Uncover the science behind physical activity, from daily routines to targeted exercises that contribute to a robust and active lifestyle.

1.　　Cardiovascular Exercise:

•　　Engage in activities like running, cycling, or swimming to boost heart health, improve circulation, and increase endurance.

2.　　Strength Training:

•　　Incorporate resistance training with weights or bodyweight exercises to build muscle strength, enhance metabolism, and support joint health.

3.　　Flexibility and Stretching:

•　　Include regular stretching exercises to improve flexibility, reduce the risk of injuries, and promote better posture.

4.　　Balance and Stability Exercises:

•　　Integrate exercises that enhance balance and stability, such as yoga or specific balance drills, to prevent falls and improve overall coordination.

5.　　Aerobic Workouts:

• Participate in aerobic exercises like dance or aerobics classes to elevate heart rate, burn calories, and boost mood.

6. Interval Training:

• Implement interval training, alternating between high-intensity and lower-intensity periods, for efficient calorie burning and cardiovascular benefits.

7. Consistency is Key:

• Establish a consistent exercise routine, aiming for at least 150 minutes of moderate-intensity or 75 minutes of vigorous-intensity exercise per week.

8. Adaptability:

• Choose activities that align with personal preferences and health conditions, making it more likely to stick to the exercise routine.

9. Mix of Activities:

• Incorporate a variety of exercises to target different muscle groups and aspects of fitness, preventing monotony and promoting overall well-being.

10. Gradual Progression:

•   Progress gradually, whether in intensity, duration, or type of exercise, to avoid overexertion and reduce the risk of injuries.

11.   Recovery Periods:

•   Allow adequate time for rest and recovery between intense workouts to prevent burnout and support muscle repair.

12.   Mind-Body Exercises:

•   Explore mind-body exercises like tai chi or Pilates to promote a holistic approach to fitness, combining physical and mental well-being.

13.   Outdoor Activities:

•   Take advantage of outdoor activities like hiking, cycling, or jogging for fresh air, exposure to nature, and added mental health benefits.

14.   Social Exercise:

•   Incorporate social elements into exercise, such as group classes or workout buddies, to enhance motivation and accountability.

15.   Posture Awareness:

• Pay attention to posture during exercise to prevent strain and promote proper alignment for maximal effectiveness.

16.   Age-Appropriate Activities:

• Choose exercises suitable for individual fitness levels and age, adapting routines as needed for optimal safety and effectiveness.

17.   Regular Health Check-ups:

• Consult with a healthcare professional before starting a new exercise regimen, especially for those with pre-existing health conditions.

18.   Hydration:

• Stay well-hydrated before, during, and after exercise to support overall bodily functions and prevent dehydration.

19.   Quality Over Quantity:

• Focus on the quality of movement rather than sheer quantity, ensuring proper form to maximize benefits and minimize the risk of injury.

20.   Celebrate Achievements:

• Acknowledge and celebrate progress and achievements in fitness goals, reinforcing positive habits and motivation.

Chapter 4: Adequate Sleep

Explore the rejuvenating benefits of quality sleep and the impact it has on overall health and longevity.

1.	Importance of Sleep:

•	Recognize sleep as a fundamental pillar of overall health, crucial for physical, mental, and emotional well-being.

2.	Recommended Duration:

•	Strive for 7-9 hours of sleep per night, as recommended by health experts, to allow the body and mind sufficient time to rejuvenate.

3.	Sleep Cycles:

•	Understand the importance of completing full sleep cycles, including both REM (rapid eye movement) and non-REM stages, for optimal restorative effects.

4.	Consistent Sleep Schedule:

•	Maintain a consistent sleep schedule, going to bed and waking up at the same time each day, to regulate the body's internal clock.

5.   Sleep Environment:

•   Create a conducive sleep environment with a comfortable mattress, pillows, and a dark, quiet room to promote uninterrupted sleep.

6.   Limit Screen Time Before Bed:

•   Reduce exposure to screens, such as phones and computers, at least an hour before bedtime to minimize the impact of blue light on melatonin production.

7.   Caffeine and Alcohol Awareness:

•   Be mindful of caffeine and alcohol intake, especially in the evening, as these substances can disrupt sleep patterns.

8.   Relaxation Techniques:

•   Practice relaxation techniques, such as deep breathing or meditation, before bedtime to calm the mind and prepare for sleep.

9.   Establish a Bedtime Routine:

•   Develop a calming bedtime routine to signal to the body that it's time to wind down, promoting a smoother transition into sleep.

10.   Physical Activity:

•	Engage in regular physical activity, but avoid vigorous exercise close to bedtime, as it may interfere with the ability to fall asleep.

11.	Avoid Heavy Meals Late at Night:

•	Refrain from consuming heavy meals late at night, allowing the digestive system to settle before bedtime.

12.	Napping Guidelines:

•	If napping, limit it to a short duration (20-30 minutes) and avoid napping too close to bedtime to preserve nighttime sleep quality.

13.	Manage Stress:

•	Implement stress-management techniques to address worries and anxieties that may otherwise interfere with falling asleep.

14.	Invest in a Comfortable Sleep Environment:

•	Choose a comfortable mattress and pillows that provide adequate support for a restful night's sleep.

15.	Natural Light Exposure:

•	Expose yourself to natural light during the day, as it helps regulate the body's circadian rhythm, promoting wakefulness during the day and sleepiness at night.

16.	Recognize Sleep Disorders:

•	If experiencing persistent sleep difficulties, consult with a healthcare professional to rule out or address potential sleep disorders.

17.	Limit Fluid Intake Before Bed:

•	Reduce fluid intake before bedtime to minimize the likelihood of waking up during the night for bathroom trips.

18.	Create a Sleep-Friendly Atmosphere:

•	Keep the bedroom cool, quiet, and dark to create an environment conducive to deep, uninterrupted sleep.

19.	Regular Check-ins:

•	Periodically assess sleep patterns and make adjustments to habits and routines to optimize sleep quality.

20.	Prioritize Sleep as Self-Care:

•	Consider adequate sleep as an essential aspect of self-care, recognizing its profound impact on physical and mental well-being.

Chapter 5: Social Connections

Dive into the significance of strong social ties, community engagement, and maintaining meaningful relationships throughout life.

1.   Inherent Human Need:

•   Acknowledge that social connections are a fundamental human need, contributing to emotional well-being and overall life satisfaction.

2.   Types of Social Connections:

•   Foster a variety of connections, including family, friends, colleagues, and community, to create a diverse and supportive social network.

3.   Quality Over Quantity:

•   Prioritize the quality of relationships over the quantity, emphasizing meaningful and authentic connections.

4.   Emotional Support:

•   Build relationships that provide emotional support, allowing for the expression of feelings, thoughts, and concerns in a safe and non-judgmental space.

5.   Physical Health Benefits:

•	Recognize the impact of social connections on physical health, as strong social ties are associated with lower rates of chronic diseases and increased longevity.

6.	Reduced Stress:

•	Engage in social interactions to reduce stress levels, as social support has been shown to mitigate the physiological effects of stress.

7.	Increased Resilience:

•	Cultivate resilience through social connections, as having a support system can help individuals cope with life's challenges more effectively.

8.	Sense of Belonging:

•	Develop a sense of belonging by actively participating in social groups or communities that align with personal interests and values.

9.	Communication Skills:

•	Hone effective communication skills to enhance the quality of social interactions and build stronger connections.

10.	Reciprocity:

•	Embrace the principle of reciprocity, offering support and care to others while also being open to receiving it when needed.

11.	Cultural and Diversity Awareness:

•	Appreciate and celebrate diversity within social circles, recognizing the richness that different perspectives and backgrounds bring to relationships.

12.	Social Bonding Activities:

•	Engage in shared activities with others to strengthen bonds, whether through hobbies, sports, or community events.

13.	Digital Connections:

•	Recognize the value of both in-person and digital connections, understanding that technology can facilitate communication but should not replace face-to-face interactions.

14.	Empathy and Understanding:

•	Practice empathy and understanding in relationships, fostering a supportive environment where individuals feel heard and validated.

15.	Conflict Resolution Skills:

• Develop skills for resolving conflicts constructively, ensuring that disagreements do not jeopardize the stability of social connections.

16. Family Connections:

• Nurture family connections, recognizing the unique significance of familial relationships in shaping one's identity and support system.

17. Friendship Dynamics:

• Understand the dynamics of friendship, acknowledging that friendships may evolve over time and embracing the positive aspects of change.

18. Community Engagement:

• Contribute to community well-being through active participation and engagement, fostering a sense of shared responsibility and connection.

19. Time Management:

• Allocate time for social connections amidst busy schedules, recognizing the importance of maintaining a balance between work and personal life.

20. Continuous Cultivation:

- Cultivate social connections continuously, investing time and effort in building and maintaining relationships as an ongoing aspect of personal growth and well-being.

Chapter 6: Healthy Aging

Learn about proactive measures to age gracefully, from skincare routines to mental agility exercises.

1.   Lifelong Learning:

•   Embrace a mindset of continuous learning and intellectual curiosity to keep the mind active and engaged.

2.   Physical Activity:

•   Incorporate regular exercise into daily routines to maintain muscle strength, flexibility, and overall physical health.

3.   Balanced Nutrition:

•   Adopt a nutrient-rich diet with a focus on whole foods to support overall health and address changing nutritional needs.

4.   Regular Health Check-ups:

•   Schedule regular health check-ups and screenings to monitor and address any potential health issues proactively.

5.   Mental Stimulation:

•   Engage in activities that stimulate the brain, such as puzzles, games, and creative pursuits, to promote cognitive health.

6.   Social Connections:

• Cultivate and maintain strong social connections to combat feelings of isolation and contribute to emotional well-being.

7. Adequate Sleep:

• Prioritize sufficient and quality sleep to support physical and mental recovery, and overall longevity.

8. Stress Management:

• Develop effective stress management techniques, such as mindfulness and relaxation exercises, to mitigate the impact of stress on health.

9. Hydration:

• Stay adequately hydrated to support various bodily functions and maintain overall well-being.

10. Preventive Measures:

• Take preventive measures, such as vaccinations and lifestyle adjustments, to minimize the risk of age-related illnesses.

11. Adaptability:

•   Embrace adaptability and resilience in the face of life changes, adjusting to new circumstances with a positive mindset.

12.   Cultivate Hobbies:

•   Cultivate hobbies and interests that bring joy and fulfillment, contributing to a sense of purpose and satisfaction.

13.   Bone Health:

•   Pay attention to bone health by incorporating calcium-rich foods, vitamin D, and weight-bearing exercises to prevent osteoporosis.

14.   Vision and Hearing:

•   Regularly check and address changes in vision and hearing to maintain a good quality of life.

15.   Regular Cognitive Assessments:

•   Consider periodic cognitive assessments to detect and address any cognitive changes early on.

16.   Medication Management:

•   Manage medications responsibly, consulting healthcare professionals for guidance on proper usage and potential interactions.

17.   Maintain a Healthy Weight:

•   Strive for and maintain a healthy weight through a combination of balanced nutrition and regular physical activity.

18.   Cultural and Social Engagement:

•   Engage in cultural and social activities to stay connected with the community and foster a sense of belonging.

19.   Sun Protection:

•   Practice sun protection measures to prevent skin damage and reduce the risk of skin cancers.

20.   Emotional Well-being:

•   Prioritize emotional well-being by addressing mental health concerns and seeking support when needed, contributing to a positive and fulfilling aging experience.

Chapter 7: Genetics and Epigenetics

Understand the role of genetics in longevity and how lifestyle choices can influence gene expression for a longer life.

Genetics:

1.   Personalized Medicine:

•   Genetic information allows for personalized medicine, tailoring treatments and interventions based on an individual's genetic profile for more effective healthcare.

2.   Disease Risk Prediction:

•   Genetic testing can identify predispositions to certain diseases, enabling proactive measures for prevention and early detection.

3.   Pharmacogenomics:

•   Understanding genetic variations helps in pharmacogenomics, optimizing drug treatments by considering an individual's genetic response to medications.

4.   Inherited Conditions Management:

•   Genetic insights assist in the management of inherited conditions, allowing for early interventions and specialized care.

5.   Family Planning Guidance:

•   Genetic information aids in family planning decisions by identifying potential genetic risks and informing choices about reproduction.

6.   Genetic Counseling:

•   Genetic counseling provides support and guidance to individuals and families in understanding and coping with genetic conditions and risk factors.

7.   Research and Drug Development:

•   Genetic research contributes to the development of new therapies and drugs, advancing medical treatments and technologies.

8.   Population Health Studies:

•   Genetic data in population health studies helps identify patterns, understand disease prevalence, and formulate public health strategies.

Epigenetics:

1.   Lifestyle Interventions:

•   Awareness of epigenetic influences encourages lifestyle modifications, such as healthy eating and stress management, to positively impact gene expression.

2.   Cancer Prevention and Treatment:

•   Targeting epigenetic changes in cancer cells provides new avenues for prevention and treatment strategies, enhancing cancer care.

3.   Environmental Adaptation:

•   Epigenetic plasticity allows cells to adapt to environmental changes, providing potential avenues for protecting against environmental stressors.

4.   Precision Medicine:

•   Incorporating epigenetic information alongside genetic data enhances precision medicine approaches, refining treatment plans for individual patients.

5.   Behavioral Interventions:

•   Epigenetic research supports the development of behavioral interventions that positively influence mental health and well-being.

6.   Aging Research:

•   Understanding epigenetic changes associated with aging opens possibilities for interventions that may slow down or reverse age-related processes.

7.   Nutritional Guidance:

•   Epigenetic influences on gene expression emphasize the importance of a balanced diet, influencing nutritional guidance for better health outcomes.

8.   Mental Health Interventions:

•   Insights from epigenetic research contribute to the development of interventions and therapies for mental health conditions, improving treatment options.

9.   Preventive Strategies:

•   Epigenetic knowledge informs preventive strategies, highlighting the role of a healthy lifestyle in promoting overall well-being and preventing diseases.

10.   Transgenerational Health:

•   Understanding transgenerational epigenetic effects enables interventions that promote health not only in the current generation but in future generations as well.

11.   Environmental Policy Considerations:

•   Epigenetic findings may influence environmental policies, emphasizing the importance of creating environments that support positive health outcomes.

12. Patient Empowerment:

• Genetic and epigenetic information empowers individuals to actively participate in their health management, making informed lifestyle choices for better outcomes.

In summary, genetics and epigenetics play pivotal roles in improving health by offering personalized insights, guiding treatment decisions, informing preventive measures, and contributing to advancements in medical research and healthcare strategies.

Chapter 8: Stress Management

Examine stress-reducing techniques and practices that contribute to a calmer, more resilient mind.

1.   Understanding Stress:

•   Recognize that stress is a natural response to challenging situations, but chronic stress can have adverse effects on mental and physical health.

2.   Identification of Stressors:

•   Identify specific stressors by assessing daily routines, relationships, work environments, and personal expectations.

3.   Mindfulness and Awareness:

•   Practice mindfulness to bring awareness to the present moment, helping to manage overwhelming thoughts and emotions associated with stress.

4.   Healthy Lifestyle Choices:

•   Adopt a balanced lifestyle with regular exercise, a nutritious diet, and sufficient sleep to enhance resilience against stress.

5.   Effective Time Management:

• Prioritize tasks and set realistic goals to manage time effectively, reducing the pressure of overwhelming workloads.

6. Social Support:

• Cultivate a strong support network by maintaining healthy relationships and seeking support from friends, family, or professionals during challenging times.

7. Relaxation Techniques:

• Incorporate relaxation techniques such as deep breathing, progressive muscle relaxation, or meditation to calm the nervous system and alleviate stress.

8. Physical Activity:

• Engage in regular physical activity, as exercise is known to release endorphins, improving mood and reducing stress.

9. Positive Thinking:

• Foster a positive mindset by reframing negative thoughts and focusing on solutions rather than problems.

10. Healthy Boundaries:

• Establish and maintain healthy boundaries in personal and professional life to prevent overwhelm and burnout.

11. Hobbies and Leisure Activities:

• Dedicate time to hobbies and leisure activities that bring joy and relaxation, providing a necessary break from daily stressors.

12. Time for Self-Care:

• Prioritize self-care activities, whether it's reading, taking a bath, or spending time in nature, to recharge and rejuvenate.

13. Humor and Laughter:

• Incorporate humor into daily life, as laughter has been shown to reduce stress hormones and improve overall well-being.

14. Cognitive Behavioral Techniques:

• Learn and apply cognitive-behavioral techniques to reframe negative thought patterns and develop healthier perspectives on stressors.

15. Work-Life Balance:

• Strive for a healthy work-life balance, setting clear boundaries between professional and personal life to prevent excessive stress from work.

16. Journaling:

• Keep a stress journal to track patterns, identify triggers, and explore effective coping mechanisms.

17.   Mindful Eating:

• Practice mindful eating, paying attention to the sensations and flavors of food, promoting a healthier relationship with eating and reducing stress-related overeating.

18.   Progressive Relaxation:

• Incorporate progressive muscle relaxation, systematically tensing and then relaxing different muscle groups, to release physical tension.

19.   Therapeutic Support:

• Seek professional help, such as counseling or therapy, to learn additional coping strategies and gain support in managing stress.

20.   Regular Check-ins:

• Regularly assess stress levels and adjust stress management strategies as needed, recognizing that personal needs and circumstances may evolve over time.

Chapter 9: Continuous Learning

Embrace the concept of lifelong learning and mental stimulation to keep the mind sharp and adaptable.

1.   Cognitive Stimulation:

•   Continuous learning keeps the brain engaged, providing ongoing cognitive stimulation that supports mental acuity and helps prevent cognitive decline.

2.   Neuroplasticity:

•   Learning new skills or acquiring knowledge fosters neuroplasticity, the brain's ability to adapt and reorganize, promoting overall brain health.

3.   Memory Enhancement:

•   Engaging in learning activities enhances memory functions, helping to retain and recall information more effectively.

4.   Problem-Solving Skills:

•   Learning cultivates problem-solving skills, enabling individuals to navigate challenges and make informed decisions for better stress management.

5.   Emotional Well-Being:

•	Continuous learning contributes to emotional well-being by providing a sense of accomplishment, purpose, and fulfillment.

6.	Reduced Risk of Cognitive Diseases:

•	Lifelong learning has been associated with a lower risk of cognitive diseases such as Alzheimer's, potentially delaying the onset of age-related cognitive decline.

7.	Adaptability:

•	Learning fosters adaptability, helping individuals better cope with change, uncertainty, and the challenges that life may present.

8.	Health Literacy:

•	Continuous learning improves health literacy, empowering individuals to make informed decisions about their health, understand medical information, and engage in preventive practices.

9.	Physical Health Benefits:

•	Intellectual curiosity and ongoing learning have been linked to better physical health outcomes, potentially reducing the risk of certain chronic conditions.

10.	Social Engagement:

•   Learning often involves social interaction, contributing to the development and maintenance of social connections, which is beneficial for mental and emotional health.

11.   Mind-Body Connection:

•   Engaging in activities that stimulate the mind through learning can positively influence the mind-body connection, promoting holistic health.

12.   Enhanced Problem-Solving:

•   Acquiring new knowledge and skills enhances problem-solving abilities, enabling individuals to address challenges and find creative solutions for improved well-being.

13.   Stress Reduction:

•   Learning can serve as a stress-relief outlet, providing a productive and enjoyable way to divert attention from stressors.

14.   Improved Sleep Patterns:

•   Mental stimulation through learning activities may contribute to improved sleep patterns, positively impacting overall health.

15.   Lifelong Curiosity:

• Cultivating a mindset of lifelong curiosity fosters a positive outlook on life, promoting mental resilience and reducing the impact of stress.

16. Career Satisfaction:

• Continuous learning can lead to career advancement and satisfaction, positively influencing mental well-being and overall life satisfaction.

17. Healthy Aging:

• Lifelong learning is associated with healthier aging, contributing to a more active and fulfilling lifestyle in later years.

18. Increased Self-Esteem:

• Accomplishing learning goals boosts self-esteem and confidence, positively affecting mental and emotional health.

19. Community Engagement:

• Learning often involves participation in community activities and organizations, fostering a sense of belonging and social support.

20. Positive Habits and Routines:

•	Learning fosters the development of positive habits and routines, supporting overall health and well-being through consistent and beneficial practices.

Chapter 10: Purpose and Passion

Explore the profound impact of having a sense of purpose and passion in life on overall well-being and longevity.

1.   Enhanced Mental Health:

•   Having a sense of purpose and pursuing passions contributes to enhanced mental health, providing a source of meaning and fulfillment.

2.   Stress Reduction:

•   Engaging in activities driven by passion and purpose can act as a powerful stress reliever, promoting relaxation and a sense of joy.

3.   Positive Outlook:

•   Having a clear sense of purpose fosters a positive outlook on life, which has been linked to better overall health and resilience in the face of challenges.

4.   Improved Emotional Well-being:

•   Pursuing passions and living with purpose is associated with improved emotional well-being, reducing the likelihood of depression and anxiety.

5.   Better Coping Mechanisms:

• Individuals with a strong sense of purpose tend to develop effective coping mechanisms, enabling them to navigate life's ups and downs with greater resilience.

6. Increased Life Satisfaction:

• Living a life aligned with one's purpose and passion often leads to increased life satisfaction, promoting a sense of contentment and fulfillment.

7. Physical Health Benefits:

• Positive emotions associated with purpose and passion can have direct physiological effects, contributing to better cardiovascular health and immune function.

8. Enhanced Cognitive Function:

• Pursuing intellectually stimulating passions can contribute to enhanced cognitive function and a lower risk of cognitive decline with age.

9. Longevity:

• Studies suggest that having a sense of purpose is associated with increased longevity, highlighting the potential impact on overall health and well-being.

10. Motivation for Healthy Habits:

• Purpose-driven individuals are often more motivated to adopt and maintain healthy habits, such as regular exercise and a balanced diet.

11. Social Connection:

• Pursuing passions often involves connecting with like-minded individuals, fostering social connections that contribute to positive mental and emotional health.

12. Reduced Risk-Taking Behaviors:

• Individuals with a clear sense of purpose are less likely to engage in risky behaviors, contributing to overall health and well-being.

13. Improved Sleep Quality:

• Passion and purpose can positively impact sleep quality, as individuals tend to experience a sense of accomplishment and peace that supports restful sleep.

14. Resilience in Adversity:

• A sense of purpose and passion acts as a buffer during challenging times, fostering resilience and helping individuals bounce back from adversity.

15. Enhanced Self-Esteem:

• Pursuing one's passions and living with purpose contributes to a positive self-image, enhancing self-esteem and confidence.

16.   Neurological Benefits:

• Engaging in activities driven by passion has been associated with neurological benefits, such as increased dopamine release, promoting a sense of reward and satisfaction.

17.   Personal Growth and Development:

• Purpose-driven living often involves continuous personal growth and development, contributing to a fulfilling and meaningful life.

18.   Immune System Support:

• Positive emotions associated with purpose and passion have been linked to a strengthened immune system, providing greater protection against illnesses.

19.   Elevated Energy Levels:

• Pursuing activities one is passionate about tends to increase energy levels, contributing to an overall sense of vitality and well-being.

20.   Holistic Health Impact:

- Purpose and passion have a holistic impact on health, influencing mental, emotional, and physical well-being, promoting a more balanced and fulfilling life.

52

15 Paths to Long Life

Chapter 11: Traditional Medicine and Alternative Therapies

Investigate ancient wisdom and alternative approaches to healthcare that have stood the test of time.

Traditional medicines:

1.   Holistic Approach:

•   Traditional medicine often adopts a holistic approach, considering the interconnectedness of the body, mind, and spirit for comprehensive health care.

2.   Cultural Context:

•   Rooted in cultural practices, traditional medicine takes into account cultural beliefs, customs, and indigenous knowledge, making it more personalized and culturally relevant.

3.   Herbal Remedies:

•   Utilization of herbal remedies, derived from plants and natural sources, is a common aspect of traditional medicine, offering potential benefits with fewer side effects.

4.   Proven Effectiveness:

•   Many traditional medicinal practices have stood the test of time, with generations of empirical evidence supporting their effectiveness in managing various health conditions.

5.   Preventive Focus:

•   Traditional medicine often emphasizes preventive measures, promoting a balanced lifestyle, dietary guidelines, and practices that support overall well-being.

6.   Integration with Modern Medicine:

•   In some cases, traditional medicine is integrated with modern medical practices, offering a complementary approach that combines the strengths of both.

7.   Patient-Centered Care:

•   Traditional medicine often involves a patient-centered approach, considering individual differences and tailoring treatments to the specific needs of the person.

8.   Cultural Heritage Preservation:

•   The practice of traditional medicine helps preserve cultural heritage and knowledge, passing down healing traditions from one generation to the next.

9.   Cost-Effective:

•   Traditional medicine can be more cost-effective than some modern medical interventions, making it accessible to populations with limited resources.

10.   Natural Healing Modalities:

•   Techniques such as acupuncture, cupping, and massage therapy are integral to traditional medicine, providing natural approaches to pain management and overall wellness.

Alternative Therapies:

1.   Mind-Body Connection:

•   Alternative therapies often focus on the mind-body connection, recognizing the impact of mental and emotional well-being on physical health.

2.   Stress Reduction:

•   Practices like meditation, yoga, and tai chi are commonly used in alternative therapies to reduce stress and promote relaxation, positively impacting overall health.

3.   Holistic Wellness:

•   Alternative therapies often address holistic wellness, considering lifestyle factors, nutrition, and emotional health as essential components of a balanced and healthy life.

4.   Complementary Approaches:

•   Alternative therapies are frequently used as complementary approaches alongside conventional medicine, providing additional options for patients.

5.   Individualized Treatments:

•   Many alternative therapies offer individualized treatment plans, recognizing that each person's health needs are unique.

6.   Energy Healing:

•   Practices like Reiki and acupuncture work with the body's energy systems, aiming to restore balance and promote healing.

7.   Mindfulness-Based Practices:

•   Mindfulness-based therapies, such as Mindfulness-Based Stress Reduction (MBSR), are utilized to improve mental health, reduce anxiety, and enhance overall well-being.

8.   Nutritional Approaches:

•   Alternative therapies often incorporate nutritional interventions, emphasizing the importance of a balanced diet for optimal health.

9.   Pain Management:

• Techniques like acupuncture and chiropractic care are used in alternative therapies for pain management, offering non-pharmacological alternatives.

10.   Cultural Variations:

• Alternative therapies encompass a diverse range of practices influenced by various cultures, allowing for a wide array of options to suit individual preferences and beliefs.

11.   Spiritual Well-being:

• Some alternative therapies, such as meditation and guided imagery, focus on spiritual well-being, providing individuals with tools to explore their inner selves.

12.   Lifestyle Modification:

• Alternative therapies often encourage lifestyle modifications, promoting habits that contribute to overall health, including regular exercise and stress management.

13.   Integrative Medicine:

• Integrative medicine combines conventional medical practices with alternative therapies, emphasizing a collaborative and comprehensive approach to health care.

14.   Biofeedback:

• Biofeedback techniques are utilized in alternative therapies to help individuals gain awareness and control over physiological processes, aiding in stress reduction and symptom management.

15.   Non-Invasive Approaches:

• Many alternative therapies are non-invasive, offering therapeutic options with minimal side effects and reduced risk compared to certain medical interventions.

16.   Enhanced Quality of Life:

• Alternative therapies are often associated with improved quality of life, providing tools for individuals to actively participate in their health and well-being.

17.   Preventive Emphasis:

• Similar to traditional medicine, alternative therapies often place emphasis on preventive measures, encouraging practices that maintain health and prevent illnesses.

18.   Empowerment and Self-Care:

• Alternative therapies empower individuals to take an active role in their health, promoting self-care practices and a deeper understanding of their bodies and minds.

In conclusion, traditional medicine and alternative therapies contribute to health improvement through diverse approaches that consider the individual, cultural context, and holistic well-being. These practices offer a range of options for individuals to explore and incorporate into their overall health and wellness strategies.

Chapter 12: Environmental Harmony

Consider the influence of a clean and sustainable environment on personal health and longevity.

1.   Clean Air and Respiratory Health:

•   Maintaining environmental harmony, including air quality, reduces the risk of respiratory issues and promotes overall lung health.

2.   Green Spaces and Mental Well-being:

•   Access to green spaces and natural environments has been linked to improved mental well-being, reduced stress, and enhanced mood.

3.   Biodiversity and Immune Function:

•   A diverse natural environment contributes to biodiversity, which, in turn, supports a robust immune system and overall health.

4.   Reduced Noise Pollution and Sleep Quality:

•   Minimizing noise pollution in the environment supports better sleep quality, positively impacting mental and physical health.

5.   Clean Water Access and Hydration:

•	Access to clean water is crucial for hydration and overall health, preventing waterborne diseases and supporting bodily functions.

6.	Natural Light and Circadian Rhythms:

•	Exposure to natural light helps regulate circadian rhythms, promoting better sleep, mood, and overall physiological function.

7.	Outdoor Exercise Opportunities:

•	An environment conducive to outdoor activities encourages regular exercise, contributing to cardiovascular health and overall fitness.

8.	Stress Reduction through Nature:

•	Spending time in natural surroundings has been shown to reduce stress levels, lower cortisol, and improve cardiovascular health.

9.	Climate Stability and Mental Health:

•	Environmental harmony, including climate stability, plays a role in mental health by reducing anxiety related to climate-related uncertainties.

10.	Natural Healing Environments:

•   Healing environments with natural elements, such as gardens or parks, can contribute to the recovery and well-being of individuals in healthcare settings.

11.   Reduced Exposure to Toxins:

•   An environmentally harmonious setting reduces exposure to toxins and pollutants, safeguarding respiratory and overall health.

12.   Enhanced Cognitive Function:

•   Green spaces and natural environments have been associated with improved cognitive function, attention, and creativity.

13.   Connection to Nature and Emotional Well-being:

•   A strong connection to nature is linked to enhanced emotional well-being, fostering feelings of peace, joy, and fulfillment.

14.   Promotion of Sustainable Practices:

•   Environmental harmony encourages sustainable practices, promoting a lifestyle that is beneficial for both personal and planetary health.

15.   Prevention of Vector-Borne Diseases:

•   Maintaining environmental balance helps prevent the proliferation of disease vectors, reducing the risk of vector-borne illnesses.

16.   Social Cohesion in Green Spaces:

•   Green spaces often serve as communal areas, fostering social interactions and a sense of community, positively impacting mental health.

17.   Reduced Urban Heat Island Effect:

•   Strategies that promote environmental harmony, such as urban greenery, can mitigate the urban heat island effect, reducing heat-related health issues.

18.   Access to Nutrient-Rich Foods:

•   Environmental harmony supports agricultural practices that provide access to nutrient-rich foods, contributing to overall health and nutrition.

19.   Preservation of Ecosystem Services:

•   Maintaining environmental harmony preserves ecosystem services, such as water purification and pollination, essential for human well-being.

20.   Promotion of Mindful Living:

• Living in harmony with the environment fosters a mindful approach to life, encouraging sustainable choices that benefit personal and collective health.

In summary, environmental harmony plays a vital role in promoting health and well-being by providing clean air and water, facilitating outdoor activities, reducing stress, and creating a supportive and sustainable living environment.

Chapter 13: Healthy Habits

Delve into small, daily habits that cumulatively contribute to a healthier and longer life.

1.   Balanced Nutrition:

•   Consuming a well-balanced diet rich in fruits, vegetables, lean proteins, and whole grains provides essential nutrients, supporting overall health and preventing nutritional deficiencies.

2.   Regular Physical Activity:

•   Engaging in regular physical activity, including aerobic exercises, strength training, and flexibility exercises, contributes to cardiovascular health, muscle strength, and overall fitness.

3.   Adequate Hydration:

•   Maintaining proper hydration supports bodily functions, aids digestion, and contributes to skin health, helping to prevent dehydration-related issues.

4.   Sufficient Sleep:

•   Prioritizing sufficient and quality sleep is crucial for physical and mental well-being, supporting cognitive function, mood regulation, and overall recovery.

5.   Stress Management:

• Implementing stress management techniques, such as meditation, deep breathing, or yoga, helps reduce the physiological and psychological impact of stress on the body.

6. Moderation in Alcohol Consumption:

• Consuming alcohol in moderation or abstaining promotes liver health and reduces the risk of alcohol-related health issues.

7. Tobacco-Free Lifestyle:

• Avoiding tobacco products, including smoking and smokeless tobacco, significantly reduces the risk of various health issues, including respiratory and cardiovascular diseases.

8. Regular Health Check-ups:

• Scheduling regular health check-ups allows for the early detection of potential health issues, promoting preventive care and timely interventions.

9. Mindful Eating:

• Practicing mindful eating involves paying attention to hunger and fullness cues, fostering a healthier relationship with food and preventing overeating.

10. Sun Protection:

•	Using sun protection measures, such as sunscreen and protective clothing, helps prevent skin damage and reduces the risk of skin cancers.

11.	Healthy Weight Management:

•	Maintaining a healthy weight through a combination of balanced nutrition and regular exercise lowers the risk of obesity-related conditions, including diabetes and heart disease.

12.	Regular Dental Care:

•	Establishing and maintaining regular dental care habits, including brushing, flossing, and dental check-ups, promotes oral health and prevents dental issues.

13.	Hygienic Practices:

•	Practicing good hygiene, including handwashing, helps prevent the spread of infections and supports overall health.

14.	Limiting Processed Foods:

•	Limiting the intake of processed and sugary foods contributes to weight management, reduces the risk of chronic diseases, and supports overall nutritional health.

15.	Cognitive Stimulation:

•   Engaging in mentally stimulating activities, such as reading, puzzles, or learning new skills, supports cognitive function and reduces the risk of cognitive decline.

16.   Social Connections:

•   Cultivating and maintaining social connections contributes to emotional well-being, reduces feelings of isolation, and supports mental health.

17.   Alcohol Awareness:

•   Raising awareness about alcohol consumption and making informed choices fosters a healthier relationship with alcohol and reduces the risk of alcohol-related harm.

18.   Mind-Body Practices:

•   Incorporating mind-body practices, such as meditation, tai chi, or yoga, supports holistic well-being by addressing both mental and physical health.

19.   Time Management:

•   Effective time management helps reduce stress, enhances productivity, and allows for the prioritization of health-promoting activities.

20.   Continuous Learning:

• Lifelong learning fosters intellectual curiosity, supports cognitive health, and contributes to a sense of purpose and fulfillment.

In summary, cultivating and maintaining healthy habits contribute to overall health and well-being by addressing various aspects of physical, mental, and emotional wellness. These habits form the foundation for a sustainable and health-conscious lifestyle.

Chapter 14: Financial Wellness

Understand the connection between financial stability and reduced stress, contributing to a longer and more fulfilling life.

1.   Reduced Stress Levels:

•   Financial stability and well-being contribute to lower stress levels, as financial concerns are a common source of stress for many individuals.

2.   Mental Health Impact:

•   Improved financial wellness positively impacts mental health, reducing the risk of anxiety and depression associated with financial struggles.

3.   Better Sleep Quality:

•   Financial stability often leads to better sleep quality, as individuals can experience reduced financial-related worries and stressors.

4.   Access to Healthcare:

•   Financial wellness enables individuals to afford healthcare services and access necessary medical treatments, contributing to overall health maintenance.

5.   Healthy Lifestyle Choices:

• Financial well-being supports the ability to make healthy lifestyle choices, including access to nutritious food, regular exercise, and preventive healthcare.

6. Reduced Risk-Taking Behaviors:

• Financial stability reduces the likelihood of engaging in risky behaviors driven by financial desperation, promoting overall health and safety.

7. Increased Physical Well-being:

• Financial wellness supports access to resources that contribute to physical well-being, including nutritious food, fitness activities, and preventive healthcare measures.

8. Improved Relationships:

• Financial stability can positively impact relationships by reducing financial stressors and promoting open communication about financial goals and responsibilities.

9. Access to Education:

• Financial wellness supports educational opportunities, enabling individuals to invest in personal and professional development, which can positively impact health.

10. Prevention of Debt-Related Stress:

•   Managing finances responsibly helps prevent debt-related stress, contributing to better mental and emotional well-being.

11.   Financial Planning for the Future:

•   Financial wellness involves planning for the future, including retirement and unexpected expenses, providing a sense of security and peace of mind.

12.   Access to Recreational Activities:

•   Financial stability allows for participation in recreational activities and hobbies, contributing to a more balanced and fulfilling lifestyle.

13.   Reduced Impact of Economic Shocks:

•   Having financial reserves and a stable financial situation reduces the impact of economic shocks, fostering resilience during challenging times.

14.   Nutritional Health:

•   Financial wellness supports the ability to afford nutritious food, contributing to better nutritional health and reducing the risk of diet-related health issues.

15.   Healthcare Decision-Making:

• Financial stability allows for more informed healthcare decision-making, as individuals can consider various treatment options without being solely limited by financial constraints.

16. Preventive Healthcare:

• Financial wellness facilitates engagement in preventive healthcare measures, including regular check-ups and screenings, promoting early detection and intervention.

17. Reduced Absenteeism at Work:

• Financially stable individuals are less likely to face absenteeism at work due to stress-related health issues, contributing to overall workplace productivity.

18. Access to Mental Health Resources:

• Financial wellness supports access to mental health resources and counseling services, providing avenues for addressing mental health concerns.

19. Reduced Physical Health Disparities:

• Financial stability can contribute to the reduction of disparities in physical health outcomes, as individuals with stable finances may have better access to healthcare resources.

20. Enhanced Quality of Life:

- Overall, financial wellness enhances the quality of life by providing the means to meet basic needs, pursue personal goals, and invest in health and well-being.

Chapter 15: Technology and Longevity

Explore how advancements in technology can support health and longevity, from wearables to personalized medicine.

Technology:

1.   Access to Health Information:

•   Technology provides easy access to health information, empowering individuals to make informed decisions about their health and well-being.

2.   Telemedicine and Remote Healthcare:

•   Telemedicine enables remote healthcare consultations, improving access to medical professionals and reducing barriers to healthcare services.

3.   Health Monitoring Devices:

•   Wearable devices and health apps allow individuals to monitor vital signs, track fitness, and manage chronic conditions, promoting proactive health management.

4.   Digital Health Records:

•   Electronic health records enhance healthcare coordination, enabling seamless communication among healthcare providers and facilitating better-informed medical decisions.

5.   Health Apps for Wellness:

•   Health and wellness apps provide tools for tracking nutrition, exercise, mental health, and sleep, promoting a holistic approach to well-being.

6.   Artificial Intelligence in Diagnostics:

•   AI technologies assist in diagnostic processes, analyzing medical data to detect patterns and aid healthcare professionals in making accurate and timely diagnoses.

7.   Precision Medicine:

•   Technology supports precision medicine approaches, tailoring treatments based on individual genetic information, improving treatment efficacy and reducing side effects.

8.   Telehealth Rehabilitation Services:

•   Telehealth platforms offer rehabilitation services, supporting individuals in recovering from injuries or surgeries from the comfort of their homes.

9.   Digital Therapeutics:

•   Digital therapeutics deliver evidence-based interventions through software, offering new avenues for managing and treating various health conditions.

10. Health Chatbots:

• AI-powered chatbots provide instant health-related information, guidance, and support, enhancing accessibility to healthcare resources.

11. Virtual Reality in Healthcare:

• Virtual reality is utilized in healthcare for pain management, mental health treatments, and simulation-based medical training, contributing to improved patient outcomes.

12. Remote Patient Monitoring:

• Remote monitoring technologies allow healthcare providers to track patients' health data in real-time, enhancing proactive care and early intervention.

13. E-Health Platforms:

• Online health platforms facilitate communication between healthcare professionals and patients, improving health literacy and patient engagement.

14. Mobile Health Clinics:

• Mobile health clinics equipped with technology bring healthcare services to underserved communities, addressing healthcare disparities.

15.   Genetic Testing and Counseling:

•   Direct-to-consumer genetic testing services provide individuals with insights into their genetic makeup, informing decisions related to health and lifestyle.

Longevity:

1.   Advancements in Medical Treatments:

•   Technological advancements contribute to improved medical treatments and interventions, extending the lifespan and enhancing the quality of life for individuals with various health conditions.

2.   Preventive Healthcare Measures:

•   Technology supports preventive healthcare measures, allowing for early detection of diseases and enabling interventions to delay or prevent the onset of age-related conditions.

3.   Personalized Health Plans:

•   Longevity-focused technologies enable the development of personalized health plans based on individual genetic, lifestyle, and health data.

4.   Regenerative Medicine:

•   Advances in regenerative medicine offer potential solutions for tissue repair and organ regeneration, addressing age-related degeneration.

5.   Anti-Aging Therapies:

•   Ongoing research explores anti-aging therapies and interventions that target cellular processes associated with aging, potentially extending lifespan and healthspan.

6.   Nutrigenomics:

•   Longevity research includes nutrigenomics, studying the interaction between nutrition and genetics to develop personalized dietary approaches that support healthy aging.

7.   Cognitive Health Technologies:

•   Cognitive health technologies focus on brain health, offering interventions and strategies to maintain cognitive function and reduce the risk of age-related cognitive decline.

8.   Biotechnology Innovations:

•   Biotechnological innovations contribute to longevity research, exploring ways to enhance cellular health and resilience.

9.   Senolytics and Senescence Research:

•	Senolytics, substances that target senescent cells, are being investigated for their potential in slowing down the aging process and promoting longevity.

10.	Lifestyle Monitoring Tools:

•	Wearable devices and health apps monitor lifestyle factors, encouraging individuals to adopt behaviors that support longevity, such as regular exercise and healthy eating.

11.	Social Connection Platforms:

•	Social connection platforms and technologies play a role in combating loneliness and promoting mental well-being, factors linked to increased longevity.

12.	Public Health Campaigns:

•	Technology aids in the dissemination of information through public health campaigns, promoting awareness about lifestyle choices that contribute to a longer and healthier life.

13.	Community Engagement Platforms:

•	Online platforms foster community engagement among individuals interested in longevity, creating spaces for information exchange, support, and collaboration.

14.	Continuous Monitoring of Health Metrics:

• Longevity-focused technologies enable continuous monitoring of health metrics, allowing for timely interventions and adjustments to support optimal health as individuals age.

15. Intergenerational Learning Platforms:

• Digital platforms facilitate intergenerational learning, allowing individuals to share knowledge, experiences, and insights related to healthy aging practices.

In summary, the intersection of technology and longevity holds significant potential for improving health outcomes. From preventive healthcare measures to advancements in medical treatments, these innovations contribute to a holistic approach to health and well-being across the lifespan.

Conclusion

"The 15 paths to long life" provides a roadmap for a vibrant, extended life by combining the wisdom of the past with the innovations of the present. Embrace these 50 paths to long life, , healthier, and more fulfilling life.